Tantric Massage

The Sensual Guide To Tantric Massage And Understanding Tantric Sex In Order To Enhance Your Sex Life

Table of Contents

Introduction 2

Chapter One: What Is Tantric Massaging? 3

Chapter Two: Tantric Massage and Sex 9

Chapter Three: Tantric Massages and Orgasms 15

Chapter Four: Is It Different For Men And Women? 21

Chapter Five: Benefits of Tantric Massages 27

Chapter Six: How Do You Know it's For You? 35

Chapter Seven: Techniques and Types 42

Chapter Eight: Keeping Tantric Massages and Sex Healthy 49

Introduction

Congratulations on downloading Tantric Massage: The Sensual Guide To Tantric Massage And Understanding Tantric Sex In Order To Enhance Your Sex Life. If you have downloaded this book, then you are either seeking the truth behind the ideologies and techniques of tantric massages, or you are wondering if it can help you overcome certain sexual dysfunctions or traumas. The good news? You have come to the right place. This book offers the truth behind the bastardized ideas of tantric massages, and it shows you how tantric massages can benefit a broad range of people. It even touches on how sexual therapies utilize them for treatment!

The answers that you seek will enable you to make the best decision for your life in regards to tantric massages, and it will even prompt you to want to use these technique in order to enhance your sexual life with your lover and partner! This book provides real-life views and scientific foundations for the benefits of tantric massages, and it explores the world of tantric massage while removing the sexual component that so many people ultimately attach to it.

I promise that when you read this book, your stereotypes will be obscure and your mind will be open to all of the possibilities and connections that both professional and personal tantric massages offer. Don't wait until the very last moment when you are struggling too much in your personal and sexual existence... Order this book now and claim what is rightfully yours!

Chapter One:

What Is Tantric Massaging?

To understand the benefits and the points of a tantric massage, one has to understand where it comes from. Tantra, as well as tantric massages, are rooted in various spiritual belief systems that originated in India (but has roots in other areas, such as Tibet and Cambodia), and are rooted in Hinduism and Buddhism. In Hinduism, there is no such thing as "instant" without somehow sacrificing an essential connection between yourself and your true nature, and that is where the length of both medicinal and erotic tantric massages is born from. Understanding how these play into both the medicinal and erotic massages will aid your understanding on how to utilize them to the best of your benefit.

Tantra is one the most underutilized branches of ancient Indian spiritual rituals. There are thousands of written texts on this idea, but it is one of the practices that keeps to the shadows. This Hindu practice dates all the way back to 5 A.D., and sprouted as a form of meditation whose aim was to elicit and maintain a state of sensuality and a calm sense of mind so that one could touch new spiritual levels. While many religions and philosophies teach either sensual or spiritual maturity, Tantra boasts of beliefs that you cannot truly have personal growth without both working in tandem with one another.

The word "tantra" is a combination of two words: *tattva* and *mantra*. *Tattva* is the science of cosmic law, *mantra* is merely a word repeated to help with concentration. So, by definition, *tantra* is the utilization of cosmic sciences to aid the focusing of the mind and body towards a higher level of spirituality.

There are many people that consider tantra to be obscene and purely sexual. During the eras in which tantra was flourishing, there were many that believed it was a form of black magic. And, while the idea of black magic no longer exists in today's modern society, the majority of the population associates sex with the word "tantra" whenever it is heard. However, the reality is that tantra is a part of the Vedic tradition, and is associated with Lord Shiva and Goddess Shakti.

The Vedic tradition is one of the oldest stratum of religious activity in India, and it is one of the major traditions that shaped and influenced Hinduism. Shiva and Shakti are the Lord and Goddess embodiments of cosmic existence, liberation, and psycho-spiritual force. Their influence on the religious connotations as well as the physical connotations stretches back thousands of years, and was born out of a need to rationalize the eternity within ourselves.

The physical manifestation of tantric massage was born out of a physical variation of tantra. It is used, quite often, as manual therapy (a way of relaxing the body). The practice rose in popularity across Asia over time, and different adaptations of the massage were born out of selfish needs that were brought forth during the act. Thus, was born the different "denominations" of tantric massaging: an American tantric massage will always be different from an East Asian one, even though they are rooted in similar histories.

The sensual side of tantric massaging was born as the practice spread west. This is, most likely, because the West had a different view of religious practices than the East. While the

East focused on spirituality and meditation to provoke inner calm, the West was focused on outer actions to atone for previous wrongdoings while reaching outward and spreading their religious beliefs elsewhere. This means that the spiritual and meditative component of tantric massages was skewed and misunderstood, and a more selfish version formed out of sheer ignorance.

Tantric massages have since started to be utilized as a medicinal technique as well as a psychology technique incorporated into practices, such as sex therapy. It is utilized as a natural prescription for people who suffer from deep anxiety issues, and has even been known to be recommended by doctors who feel the need to treat one's depression with something other than medication. But, do not get this form of tantric massage confused with the erotic tantric massage. While the two are rooted in the same spiritual practices, they have two very different outcomes and implementation styles. This type of tantric massage therapy is relaxing and pleasuring the body, but aiding in balancing the brain by promoting certain chemical reactions that aid in relaxation and comfort.

The main focus of a tantric massage is creating and maintaining the balance between male and female energies (Shiva and Shakti). It is utilized to promote balance, a healthy mindset, and a relaxed state of being.

Erotic tantric massages are highly sensual and are rooted in the idea of teaching individuals (primarily men) how to embrace their sexuality. The art of tantra focuses on massage movements that are specifically designed to stimulate physical arousal, but prolong this pleasure by delaying orgasm alongside proper breathing techniques. An erotic tantric massage combines the balancing of the body's energies with sharing mutual pleasures with another human being, therefore promoting healthy emotions and attractions. An erotic tantric massage is also a journey of learning with your partner, specifically teaching a male the ability to maintain a high arousal state that ends in a climax without ejaculation.

Tantra, the religious belief that his was born from, is really a path to self-actualization. It is rooted in the idea of safe self-exploration by taking specific actions that reveal our deepest thoughts and bringing them to the surface to aid in understanding ourselves better. By knowing yourself better through these actions, you can then condition yourself in whatever you wish, influencing your own actions instead of relying on what you were conditioned with as a child. Nothing that you do is really you, it is a by-product of everything you experienced as a child. Tantra holds the belief that, by utilizing its techniques as they should be, anyone can re-influence themselves despite how they grew up.

Tantra was used as a form of self-healing. It was used for those who grew up in less-than-ideal conditions who were robbed of their ability to influence their lives as they saw fit. While the sexual aspect of tantra has been deemed normal, it is not where its roots lie. Over time, the practice became bastardized into the purely erotic form that connotes it today, and many people who "practice" tantric massages usually know nothing of the religious practices and practical necessities from which it is born.

Massage therapists who practice tantric massages for relaxation and medicinal purposes believe that these types of massages can help clear our bodies of accumulated toxins. The belief is that it promotes healing, regeneration of healthy cells, promotes positive chemical reactions in the brain that reverberate throughout the body, and aid in reconnecting us with our surrounding spiritual energies. And, they aren't wrong. There is a lot of scientific studies out there on the medicinal foundations of massaging, and the sheer length of tantric massages, medicinal or otherwise, would promote those positive side effects for a much longer time than a regular massage.

This idea that we are all filled with the same energy as the earth surrounding us is what leads Tantric's to believe that, when we disassociate ourselves from the world around us, this disconnection leaves us damaged and unbalanced in the way of our mindset, our body's health, and our anxieties. Tantra complete rejects the self-deniance that people live in from day-to-day. They spit upon the guilt that people are imposed to feel when someone's sexual and sensual needs rise to the surface, and promote attentive pro-activeness to solving these issues rather than avoidance.

As one grows, blockages will always form in our path. Tantric's believe that those blockages need to be completely cleared out rather than just steered around in order to address and put into practice a unifying bond between our physical bodies and our spiritual energies. Think of it as a kinked water hose: if you fold it in half, you only acquire a reduced water supply. In return, as you begin to water your garden, it takes you much longer to feed your plants what they need in order to grow the way they should. This, in turn, requires more of your time in order to fulfil. The same goes for your body: if you have blockages that are reducing the flow of your spiritual energy, when it comes time for your energies to aid you in an important task, such as growing and fulfilling things around you, it will take you a much longer time to fulfil those tasks because your "hose is kinked."

They believe that, instead of punching a different hold into the already-kinked hose, you should just release the kink.

Tantric massages, both medicinal and erotic, hold various benefits for the mind, the body, and the soul. They impact men and women differently on a level that promotes physical healing, sexual satisfaction, and emotional awareness. The roots of its practice are embedded deeply in the religious roots of the Indian and Tibetan cultures, and the bastardization of it as it spread across the West needs to be addressed: Tantra, and the practices that come along with it, are not just for sexual satisfaction. Tantra is used to combine two distinct forces, physical growth and sensual satisfaction, to bring about self-awareness and self-confidence while promoting self-sufficiency and a bond with the earth and energies around you. Tantric sex is not just for sexual release. It is for healing, guiding, and taking control of your body and mind in ways you have not discovered yet.

This book will delve into the differences between techniques of tantric massages, how science can back up the medicinal form of these massages, how the erotic form of these massages actually works, and the overall benefits that come as a result of practicing this religious art form, whether you mean for them to happen or not.

Chapter Two:

Tantric Massage and Sex

A tantric massage is a very sensual, close, meditative experience with one's partner. A tantric massage not only consists of the physical massage, but it includes meditative and closeness exercises leading up to the sensual touches and sensations. This massage includes many different techniques from different schools of thought from massage therapy. It pulls elements from yoga, sexual therapy, and even bioenergetics. The first time a "tantric massage" was branded as such an activity was in the 1980s by Andro Andreas Rothe. He established the first professional Tantra institute in Germany in 1977, and the modernized experience took off from there. In a professional tantric massage (that does not utilize the massaging motions to produce an orgasmic experience), the client plays a very passive role in the entire process. Just as a "normal" massage would, the client is simply lying back, relaxing, and allowing the masseuse to do what he or she does. The entire process combines elements of well-being, relaxation, and therapeutic confrontation of sexual issues, should the client have been recommended by a sex therapist.

The purest definition of a tantric massage does not require a sexual exchange of any kind. It has been utilized as a form of sexual therapy for as long as legitimate sexual therapy has been around, and has had many positive results brewed from its existence. While the idea of tantra and "tantric expression" is rooted in Eastern religions, the purely sexual aspect is rooted in the works of Carl Jung and Wilhem Reich, who believed that sexual expression and fulfilment were necessary in maintaining a positive and constant personal growth. However, despite the sexual aspects that are outlawed in various countries, places such as Switzerland and Germany have attempted to make erotic tantric massages (complete with the orgasmic ending) a taxable service.

The erotic and more sensual forms of tantric massaging is the strict purpose of using this massage to achieve orgasm. This type of massaging specifically targets erogenous zones and nerve endings to help stimulate, heighten sexual senses, and eventually achieve the ultimate feeling of pleasurable release. For women, the two most popular focal points of an erotic tantric massage are the breasts and the pubis. For men, it is their buttocks and genital regions. This includes the massaging of areas such as the inner thigh, the crest of the hip joint, atop the pubis bone, and even the area around one's belly button.

The idea behind a true erotic tantric massage is connection and taking one's time. It is common for erotic massages to be used as foreplay to a grander scheme, but tantric sex isn't the foreplay, it is the actual show. Those who utilize the slow, languid movements of a tantric massage usually couple it with basic positions, strong eye contact, and meditative conversation. This meditative conversation is usually spoken lowly and within close contact of one another, and utilizes praises and compliments to enhance the confidence and connection that one is trying to acquire with their partner.

There is another component to tantric massages, both for therapeutic purposes and for erotic purposes, and that is the concept of "energy work." This idea stems around bringing your emotions to the surface. For those that are undergoing sexual therapy, it is usually to help them cope with traumatic sexual experiences while regaining control of their personal sexual desires. For those who are using it for more erotic purposes, the goal is to bring your true feelings for your partner to the surface so that you can acknowledge an unspoken truth between the two that culminates into a mutual pleasurable experience.

A tantric massage focuses mainly on stimulating the specific nerves located on or near someone's sexual organs. The belief is that this constant and slow stimulation creates new pathways of sensation that ricochet through one's body and, ultimately, to the brain. In a religious context, this was to broaden the mind to things not understood by someone who didn't have a clarity of mind. In a more sexual context, this simply means that the person receiving the massage experiences a new kind of sexual sensation that doesn't involve rapidly climbing to what they ultimately want. The focus is on removing the block that society has conditioned many to believe, resulting in guilty thoughts when it comes to sexual desires. As these blocks are removed, more sexual energy can flow through the "channels" of one's body, and it frees individuals up to be more self-expression in the world because of the release they experience.

Those that teach the basics of tantric massages say that there are a few things that you can do every single time to enhance the experience. The actual part of the massage involves lightly touching the skin with flowers, fabrics, feathers, ice, fingertips, and even hot wax. Beginning with a gentle touch is imperative, and slowly making your way to fuller and longer strokes allows your partner to be able to slowly slip into a relaxed state of mind. This enables them to open their mind to new sensations while simultaneously slowing themselves down. In a rushed world, intimacy feels rushed as well. Tantric massages aim to slow that down and redefine how intimacy is framed.

Lying face down enables the person to open their bodies and minds to various sensations, and the act of closing one's eyes allows them to look inwardly at how each stroke, caress, and long, languid stroke is affecting their bodies internally. It creates a sense of self-awareness while creating a trusting connection between you and your partner. The start begins at zones that are not considered erogenous, such as the neck, feet, and hands. Then, as their bodies relax and they begin to slip into a trusting and freeing zone, the masseuse begins to move their strokes towards zones that are considered sexual, such as the bottom, genitals, and inner thighs.

When ample time has been spent on the back, then the client slowly turns over, syncing up their breaths with the movements of their body, and their awakened skin is awarded with soft touches. Again, the massage resets, focusing on zones that are seemingly non-erogenous before working to zones that are.

Constant feedback from the masseuse is necessary. They are encouraged to keep reminding their partner to breathe in fully, stay present, and relax. These parts of the massages, even though erogenous zones are being stimulated, do not end in orgasm. The purpose of the massage is to slowly build the body to that point. This is simply about providing trusting pleasure. This, in turn, can lead to moments that create orgasm, such as making love or mutual masturbation techniques. However, there are some couples that switch roles, and when both have been relaxed and fulfilled inwardly, they lie in each other's arms and share their feelings in light conversation.

It is encouraged, if love making does enter the picture, to not be rushed. Penetration happening naturally, as opposed to simply "going for it," is encouraged because it follows the trend already set forth by the couple, and it allows for true and unadulterated sensations to flow through these new energy channels that now exist between the body's pleasure centres and the brain. No effort should go into any sort of penetration. If there is effort, then it has not been done right.

There are ways to connect before employing a tantric massage, and they are outlined very clearly by many teachers and institutions across the world. A traditional tantric pose, called the "Yab Yum" pose. This pose consists of the male partner (or the more dominant partner) sitting cross-legged on the floor. Then, the female (or the less dominant partner) sits down on top of him with his/her legs facing him. This pose can be done clothed or naked, depending on how the tantric massaging and erotic motions have progressed. The two partners then embrace and synchronize their breathing with one another. This allows one's bodies to tune into their partner's, and an energy-fusing embrace emerges, connecting the two bodies spiritually.

Another tip that tantric professionals give is looking into the eyes of one's partner. The eyes have constantly been considered the gateways to the soul, and there have even been scientific studies done that state that when you gaze into someone's eyes for at least 20 seconds, there is a chemical reaction in the brain that takes place. This chemical reaction enables a feeling of trust to take place, thereby creating a closer connection between the two individuals. Utilize this chemical reaction to your advantage. The synchronizing of your breath with your partner's is still encouraged during this stage because it enhances the connection you are building with one another.

There are other aspects, such as music and meditative thought processes, that can enhance the experience before the touching ever beings. The purpose of a tantric massage is not to chase an orgasm. Its purpose is to create a feast of the pleasure that comes with orgasm instead of taking bite-sized pieces of it selfishly. It blends techniques of meditation and yoga to create a deep connection with someone that culminates to a slow, guided, pleasurable experience. A tantric massage does not always end in an orgasm, but it should always end with a deeper connection and understanding of the person that has enacted the experience alongside you.

Tantric massages and sex do not always go hand-in-hand. They can be used therapeutically with no orgasm involved, and they can be utilized for emotional and sexual therapy purposes, which have solid grounds in new theories being raised in psychology today. Either way, a tantric massage is a highly emotional experience whose root belief consists of the understanding that the body cannot fully function or enjoy the world around it without fulfilling all aspects of our body's needs. Tantra recognizes sexual desires as an innate need, and works to fulfil that desire by redefining what it means to the average person. A tantric massage is just one way to accomplish that goal, and, if done correctly, can result in a newfound way to explore sexual intimacy, emotional intimacy, and redefine what it means to be mentally intimate with someone.

Chapter Three:

Tantric Massages and Orgasms

A therapeutic tantric massage and an erotic tantric massage have very little differences. Both can bring a person to orgasm, both are intimate moments within intimate settings, and both are utilized (in part) for relaxation purposes. The main difference is the relationship between the receiver and the masseuse, and the venue where it is performed.

For some, tantric massages do not end in orgasm. But, for those that do, there is a specific way in which this is achieved, and it is said to be the most effective way to relieve stress, open energy channels from the pubis to the brain, and to orgasm. It begins with setting the mood: relaxing scents such as lavender, flickering candles with no odours (or odours that do not counteract the scents wafting within the room), and a comfortable place for the recipient of said massage to relax. Unscented oil works best if you already have incense and scented candles going in the room, and the oil helps to reduce skin-to-skin traction.

Once this setting is complete, a head-to-toe massage commences. Beginning at the head, you slowly work your way down the body, massaging every single place available: the scalp, the ears, the cheeks. Usually people start out lying on their stomach, so the masseuse works their way down slowly, making sure to pay great attention to the buttocks. Once the masseuse reaches the feet, each individual toe is massaged before the client is prompted to turn over. Then, the hands slowly work their way up each leg, massaging the inner thigh so close that the backs of the masseuse's hands brush against the vagina (or penis) of the client.

Then, that area is skipped over to finish the rest of the frontal full-body massage. The masseuse slowly works up the stomach, paying great attention to the breasts, and when they make their way back up to the scalp of the recipient, then they turn their attentions between the legs of the client. Each individual part of the vagina (or penis) of the client is massaged, and while orgasm is usually achieved, sometimes it is not. In an erotic massage, when attention is turned towards the genital area, mouths usually come into play in order to induce orgasm. In a professional atmosphere, once each part of the genitalia on the client has been massaged, the massage is over, whether or not an orgasm has been achieved.

In a professional environment, the mouth of the client never touches the recipient's body. In an erotic sense, the couple has much more leeway with that type of action depending on their comfort level with one another. However, the ideal tantric massage takes anywhere between two and three hours (in a professional setting, a half an hour is devoted to a pre-massage consultation and another half an hour is devoted at the end to a post-massage conversation), is done slowly and gently (with varying degrees of pressure depending solely on the recipient's wants and needs), and requires a relaxing, intimate atmosphere in order to gear both of the participant's mindsets and bodily energies towards the task at hand.

There are even workshops dedicated to teaching individuals and couples on how to properly give and receive tantric massages. While the focus of these workshops isn't achieving orgasm, they teach that the foundation of a tantric massage (whether erotic or not) is not merely just to chase an orgasm. They teach tantric massages and its correct techniques as a way to achieve the ultimate form of relaxation, a deep connection between one's mind and one's body, a deep sense of self-actualization.

In these workshops, many people are drawn by the same tired ideals: treating the body as just an object, making love to nothing more than an idea, the inevitable struggle to reach orgasm because of that disconnection from your body, and the ultimate feeling of being disconnected from their partners. People come to these workshops wanting more out of an area of their life that is no longer fulfilled. They state that they feel bogged down in these sexually-repressed feelings, and that they believe that is what is holding them back in their everyday lives.

However, what is quickly discovered within these workshops is that Tantric principles aren't just applicable to sex and sexual adventures. The qualities that are taught) like mindfulness, gratitude and reverence) enhance every other aspect of life and how one lives it. In these tantric massage workshops, the aim of is not orgasm. That is a very important point that needs constant reinforcement in the world of Tantra and tantric massages. Many people view it as alternative way to chase an orgasm that they haven't attempted with their partners yet. True and real tantric massages have nothing to do with reaching orgasm.

Respecting one's individual sexual energy and learning how to take control of it can be healing for both men and women. For example, strengthening someone's pelvic floor muscles via Kegel exercises, or even the use of jade eggs, is incredibly important for women because it allow them to use sexual energy safely, and can even aid in other physical ailments such as an uncontrollable bladder. Jade eggs are essentially a smooth, egg-shaped object that is inserted into the yoni (the tantric word for "vagina") and held there by clenching one's Kegel muscles in order to keep it stable. Think of it as strength and resistance training for the muscles that control the walls of a woman's vagina.

In these workshops, lingam (the tantric word for "penis") massages are also taught. They are not taught on actual penises, however. In one particular workshop, oil and phallically-shaped vegetables were involved. However, prior to the appearance of any vegetables, the masseuse has to take the time to ensure a warm, comfortable, relaxing, and safe environment for all parties involved. Some people enjoyed the aspect of cushions and candles, some enjoyed the sounds of running water and refreshing smells, and some even enjoyed simply laying on a bed in dim lighting. But, after the area is set up for ultimate relaxation and everyone has become comfortable, then the full body massage begins. There is constant check-up on the recipient that includes reminders of breathing techniques and inquires about hand pressure, and the entire process occurs over a period of hours.

There are certain massaging motions that are taught and utilized within practice, like the "Tickle and Scratch" and the "Wax On, Wax Off," but once you harness your partner's sexual energy within your fingertips, you can then move it around the body and create a unifying experience between the two of you. This process can go on for as long as both parties wish, and at no point in time is the point ever orgasm. However, if this takes place during the workshop, it's alright.

Many people proclaim that, after these workshops and professional massages, that their bodies feel more relaxed. They boast of a better sex life, and one that ultimately becomes more in tune with the true wants and needs of the body rather than the one that is only temporary. Tantra, and the tantric massage, are tools and beliefs that are preached and taught to harness the energy within yourself as well as with your partner so that your energies (and bodies) can synchronize. It is about achieving a closeness and connection not normally found in the usual encounter you have with someone (whether it is sexual or not) and it focuses on the benefits of self-realization and finding the truth deep within yourself.

But, a tantric massage isn't just to enhance everything prior to the peak of a sexual experience. A tantric massage, when utilized correctly, connects your body to a never-ending spring of relaxation and peace that can last for hours after the fact. Within the religious beliefs of Tantra and tantric sex, sexual love and the fulfilment that comes with giving that part of someone's life what it truly needs is considered a sacrament. Through the act of sex and the slow-growing pleasure that comes with it, the two people involved become one with each other and with the universe's energies. The unblocking of new channels and the enlarging of existing energy channels that is derived from the slow, relaxing massage enhances the idea of a full-body orgasmic experience, which isn't to be confused with an actual orgasm.

A full-body orgasmic experience is when one releases the tension, guilt, and apprehension that comes with the conditioning of deeming sexual acts "uncouth." By releasing these blockages, more efficient energy pathways are opened up between the body, the soul, and the mind, and the releasing experience results in a prolonged effect of internal orgasm. Instead of a quick and localized genital stimulation, there is the experience of subtle and prolonged pulsations and vibrations throughout the body that cause you to feel as if you are melting into your partner. This, in turn, stimulates one's brain cells and creates a sort of "bridge" between the left and right hemispheres. By being able to fuse and access the best of both hemispheres, the achievement results in a prolonged experience of ecstasy that the body, mind, and heart all participate in.

Statistics tell us that the average sex session between two individuals is 20 minutes, including foreplay, and that the average female orgasm lasts for 15 seconds while the average male orgasm lasts for only 10. However, once someone can learn to manipulate the external pleasurable experience of an orgasm (should that be one's end goal with a tantric massage) and revert it internally, pulling it through different organs of the body, there are many individuals, including Sting and Woody Harrelson, that have boasted of 30 minute orgasmic experiences.

Tantric massages and orgasms have a complicated relationship. A tantric massage, whether professional or not, never has the purpose of an orgasm. However, the types of stimulations and relaxations that occur usually enable the recipient the approach and reach orgasm faster, and with more ease, than they are used to. Then, it becomes a matter of personally breaking down why that reaction took place. This beginning journey of self-actualization is what Tantra, and tantric massages, is all about. The connection between partners, and between them and the universe, open up the mind to spiritual realities and energies not tapped into because of the lack of attention they were giving to their minds and the overload of attention they were giving to something that was temporary.

Tantric massages seek to give those that want control of their bodies a way to get back in touch with themselves, and it is that connection with themselves that opens them up to deeper connections with others, whether or not the connection is sexual.

Chapter Four:

Is It Different For Men And Women?

Men and women experience sensations differently. Part of it is hormonally-based, and part of it is emotionally-based. The mere fact that they experience things differently means that different things will result from Tantra and tantric massages. Research indicates that things such as pain, happiness, and even orgasm are experienced differently, and hardwired differently, within a male and female's brain.

Research gives us more evidence every year that male and female brains have different ways of processing emotion. Past research has proved that women experience higher levels of emotional stimulation due to hormonal and chemical reaction than men. But now? A new, massive-scale study done at the University of Basel has brought to light that gender differences in emotional processing are linked to sex (and its variations) in memory and brain activity. The Basel researchers conducted an experiment that would ultimately determine whether or not women innately performed better on memory tests than men. Their basis for justification was due to the way they process emotional information chemically. The researchers found 3,400 test participants to participate, and the task included being exposed to images of emotional content. Via measuring different chemical reactions and electrical brain reactions, they found that women rated the images as more emotionally stimulating than men, especially when it came to negative images. Their baseline was presenting the men and women with emotionally neutral imagery, where both men and women responded similarly.

After the exposure to the images and the ratings of the images were recorded, the participants were instructed to complete a memory test. Overall, the female participants could recall significantly more of the images than the male participants, and the women also proved to have an enhanced ability to recall the positive images. This entire thing suggests that the massively-skewed differences in emotional processing, as well as the ability to recall one emotion over another, are due to mechanisms within the brain and the brain's memory capacities that are gender determined.

But not only that, fMRI scans from over 700 of those participants provide visible proof that backs up claims to a woman's innate ability to react more to negative emotional images. The scans show that these reactions to outer stimuli are linked with increased activity of motor regions of the brain. Many other previous studies have also suggested and proven that women display more intense facial and motor reactions to negative emotional stimuli than men. In the fMRI data patterns, the parts of the brain stimulated are clearly seen, and can be compared side-by-side to those of males while the differences are analysed with the naked eye.

It is these types of findings that begin to explain why women are more susceptible to debilitating depression, major anxiety disorders, and post-traumatic stress disorder. The theory is that if they experience regular emotional responses more intensely, then they would also experience irregular emotional responses more intensely. These emotional processing responses that seem to be sex-specific are not only valuable in improving medical treatment options for emotional and mental disorders, it also means that things that evoke strong emotions, such as tantric massages, are more strongly felt for women than men.

However, this does not mean that men cannot experience intense sensations and emotions via tantric massages. It just means that they experience it differently than women.

Just like emotions, men and women also experience pain differently. Dr. Andreas Sander-Kiesling found at the Medical University of Graz found that, directly after surgeries like heart and shoulder surgery, experienced more pain directly after an operation than women. However, women were found to have higher pain levels than men after routine surgeries, such as biopsies. This leads Dr. Sander-Kiesling to hypothesize that this physical response is also rooted emotionally, with women connecting more pain to things that generate more emotion (such as biopsies for cancers that affect their time with their families, and even abortions that invade them physically). These greater anxieties on how they will affect their overall quality of life induce greater anxieties, which are already heightened by sex-specific chemical reactions. This hypothesis, if proven correct, provides a foundational understanding of why women and men experience pain differently.

And this is what brings us to the real question: do men and women experience orgasm differently? If physical sensations, like pain after surgeries, can be enhanced merely by the emotional component behind the reason for the surgery, then it is possible that women experience different orgasms from men on an emotional level and not just a physical one. It's a fair question, and one that needs some specific attention to answer.

Minus the fact that men and women have different physical parts that react in different physical ways, an orgasm also affects the brain. And, because we have proven that the male and female brain operate differently from one another, then it is very possible that orgasms that register physically and chemically can also be altered by the different emotional states of the two parties in play.

In order to measure orgasms on a physical level, brain scans to measure cerebral blood flow in men and women have been utilized. These brain scans have been taken by willing participants in various studies, both during genital stimulation, during orgasm, and directly after. An orgasm is a physical sensation, and any physical sensation that happens in the body is manipulated and caused by the brain.

Janniko Georgiadis (at the University of Groningen) utilized PET scans (positron emission tomography) to measure these three different points of pleasure during genital stimulation and the reactions after. What was found were significant differences electrical activation patterns not only during arousal but during the orgasm itself. The immediate response was that the differences in electrical activity could simply be due to the fact that what stimulates a penis might not always stimulate a clitoris, though that is not believed by everyone.

Various other studies have taken different measurement practices, measuring things such as frequency, intensity, and the duration of pelvic muscle contractions during orgasm (which are measured with a pressure sensitive anal probe). These tests were done on willing participants who were performing masturbation rituals, and the final results showed many similarities in these contraction patterns between men and women. This gives further proof to the theory that, while the physical responses can align all they want, the emotional responses that chemically take place in the brain can change the sensation of the orgasm, depending on the gender of the participant.

Near-identical responses to physical sexual stimulation, according to psychology Alan Fogel, has a very good reason that is based in our basic evolution. The theory is that these shared experiences that have emotionally intense context enhance a couple's connection in a bodily sense. For example, if we see someone crying, we empathize and feel sad for them. If we see someone scared, we empathize and feel fear for their safety alongside them. Likewise, when we observe someone else having an orgasm, no matter what gender, it enhances the desire, and readiness for, experiencing our own orgasm.

To test this theory, many studies reverted back to the fMRI scans utilized throughout various studies, and while they show significant similarities between genders and how they electrically produce orgasms within the brain, they are also exposing subtle differences that make massive changes.

Part of these series of studies involved taking the fMRI's of men and women who were stimulated by each other and compared them to the fMRI's taken when measuring men and women during self-stimulation. They took a look at differences in blood flow, electrical activity, which areas of the brain were activated as a response to the stimulation, and even how the pelvic muscles reacted during orgasm. What these findings found was that women experienced significantly more activation of the part of their brain that is responsible for processing sensations when they were with someone than when they were alone.

The theory behind this difference is that the emotional connection that comes with stimulation alongside a partner plays a role in how they physically and mentally experience an orgasm. If all of that is proven to be correct, than men and women do, in fact, experience orgasm differently.

Tantric massages are utilized to tap into unused energies, both mentally and emotionally. Because of the fact that women experience pain and pleasure more intensely because of their gender-specific hardwiring, this means that there is a basis for women experiencing tantric massages differently than men. This does not mean that the difference is more pleasurable, or somehow more intense, than the experience that men have, it just means that there is a physical difference in how orgasms and tantric massages are received emotionally, physically, and chemically.

Think of it this way: if you put two people side-by-side who have lost someone close to them in their families, you will be able to find different physical reactions by observing them. One might cry more than the other, or one might talk considerably more about them than the other. One of them might try to hold back their tears and swallow more to keep them at bay, and one might not even shed tears until they are alone to cope by themselves. These differences in reactions don't mean that they are feeling different levels of sadness. Quite the opposite, they are both hurting and grieving intensely inside. It just means that, chemically (and by being conditioned by their surroundings as children), it is producing different physical reactions.

No matter the physical, mental, or emotional reaction, tantric massages are all supposed to do the same thing: take the emphasis off temporary physical intimacy and incorporate true, and elongated, feelings of inward emotional intimacy for your partner. It is supposed to enhance and bring together two souls that wish to combine themselves with the energies of the universe in order to fulfil every innate part of them that begs for sustenance.

And those needs that are begged for are not gender-specific.

Chapter Five:

Benefits of Tantric Massages

Tantra, and all of its beliefs, have been practiced for over 9,000 years. Way back in the Himalayan Mountains in India, religious leaders fully believed that sexual ritual, as well as fulfilling the sexual aspect of the human form, was the ultimate path to a higher form of liberation and connection with the energies of the spiritual world. In today's world, the teachings of Tantra are taken and translated into a full-body experience that doesn't just hinge on the fulfilment of sexual desires and wishes. This traditional message is subsequently heightened by utilizing breathing exercises and genital stimulation (neither of which were used with the religious leaders of the olden days). Not only is the massage benefiting in a relaxing manner, it can also bring about ways to cope with sexual trauma by slowly tackling the PTSD of the event in a mild, trusting, and controlled environment.

A tantric massage relaxes every single part of the body. It doesn't just address an aching back and stiff shoulders, it tackles every single muscle in the body. The massage consists of two to three hours of massaging each and every muscle, both big and small, to release that deep-seated stress that sits in the small crevices of the body. This relaxation doesn't just become physical, it ends up manifesting in a spiritual manner that relaxes the soul as well. After all, 80% of people who experience a tantric massage for the first time end up being returning customers.

Not only does a tantric massage revolve around relaxation, there are also specific breathing techniques that the client is talked through during the massage. These breathing techniques help to centre the mind, calm the soul, and promote inward reflection and self-awareness. For those that are slowly overcoming sexual trauma, these breathing techniques are used to slow down the natural adrenal response that comes with PTSD-driven emotions and memories, and gives them a viable method for self-calming their body during the massage. The breathing enhances the overall experience and gives control back to those who feel that they have lost it.

A tantric massage can provide a state of emotional healing as well. It isn't just the physical attributes of the massage that encourages people to come back, it is also the healthy emotional promotion that draws them back as well. Learning to lean back and receive that kind of pleasure with absolutely no contest of reciprocation is a revalidation of self-worth. This can impact the overall state of happiness of the client, and it can slowly help teach someone that receiving this type of "gift" (as in, receiving the "gift" of relaxation and happiness) does not have to come with the stress of having to reciprocate it. It teaches people to slowly accept the happiness that is due to them without having to create imaginary stressors based on how they will be perceived if the actions aren't reciprocated.

However, the pleasurable aspect can't be overlooked. The sheer enjoyment that comes from feeling every single muscle in your body relaxing can be positively overwhelming, and the thrill of the emotional and spiritual balance can become intoxicating. There is also the physical pleasure that is sometimes brought with tantric massages (in the form of orgasm) that can bring on a heightened sense of relaxation and happiness. Keep in mind, however, that orgasm is not the ultimate goal. It never is with a tantric massage. The spiritual, emotional, and physical relaxation and binding your energies with the universe is the ultimate goal.

A tantric massage can also help people to curb impulses. The breathing techniques that are taught and acquired during tantric massages can also be utilized to control other aspects of the client's life, such as food cravings and premature ejaculation. These natural human impulses can be controlled, just like in the tantric massage, because the breathing techniques promote the re-focusing of one's mind.

And, as if that isn't enough, the mere intensity of the massage and the attention that each of your muscles obtains, the promotion of blood circulation can contribute to many blatant health benefits. Color can return to the skin, organs can begin to function more efficiently, things such as eyesight and hearing can become better, and even chronic headaches can be treated with better blood circulation that a tantric massage can provide.

A tantric massage can provide a massive amount of benefits. Not only does it have individual benefits that many massage don't tackle, it also tackles the original benefits of the massage in the first place! Things such as pain management that comes with extreme muscle tension and fatigue are addressed with the total body attention that a tantric massage can provide. The elongated average time of the massage ensures that every single ache and pain that the client is experiencing is fully and completely taken care of.

Also, many people who seek out regular massages for the treatment of migraines and headaches will find the same type of treatments within a tantric massage. And, because a tantric massage promotes the massaging of every single muscle in the body, better blood circulation can occur long after the client has left the appointment, which means that the effects of the massage last longer than that of a regular massage.

However, probably one of the best benefits that is chronically raved about are the sleep improvements that tantric massages spawn. The overall quality of sleep is improved because the body is more relaxed, blood circulation is better, and the pain management that a tantric massage can bring works its way into how your body seeks out sleep, providing an uninterrupted state of sleep as well as a deeper state of sleep.

The wonderful thing is that absolutely everyone can benefit from a tantric massage. Practicing and learning about Tantra can open up so many different doorways that lead to both an increase in sexual healing and desire as well as promote a state of self-awareness that not many ever achieve within their lifetime. The health benefits are overwhelming, and many have professed that they prefer it to medicinal treatments of certain health issues (such as general aches, pains, and headaches). A tantric massage can open up someone's mind and soul to an immense connection between the energies of the world and the physical energies raging within their bodies, and it can create an overwhelming sensation that roots them to the ground and promotes an overall positive state of mind.

Tantric massage has also been finding its way into the medicinal world. While it isn't a conclusive treatment for anything, the benefits that have been proven can also be rooted in other health issues. For example, the promotion of better blood circulation can lead to aiding in treatment of inflammatory diseases. The promotion of self-awareness and breathing exercises can calm and slow down the mind, which can aid people who have been diagnosed with anxiety disorders and A.D.H.D.

With the promotion of relaxation and the reduction of stress that comes with a tantric massage, benefits such as aiding in digestion and hormone imbalances can also be tackled within a few sessions. While a doctor will never prescribe one for you, the benefits that have been proven with regular massages translate in a deeper aspect to tantric massages, which is why so many people can proclaim so many different benefits.

Tantra proclaims that the reason it can aid in all of these mental and physical disabilities is because a tantric massage can relieve energy blockages and readdress energy imbalances within the body. During a tantric massage, the belief is that there are only two things that cause physical pain within the body: a blockage of the flow of blood and the blockage of the flow of energy. Tantra focuses on promoting better blood circulation through deep breathing and meditation, and it focuses on relieving energy blockages through relaxation, circular massaging, and strict attention to every single part of the body.

With a tantric massage, no part of the body is neglected (unlike a regular massage, which promotes relaxation as well as physical purity) and every single atom of the client's body is addressed in much the same way. This promotes a physical cohesiveness that translates into a spiritual cohesiveness that is promoted within.

While there is a sexual energy focus as well, the point is that this is not the main component of a tantric massage. The sexual energy that is addressed within a tantric massage does not have an end goal of sexual pleasure. The point is that sexual energy is released within the body, aids in energetic circulation by relieving guilt-ridden and stressed blockages throughout the body, and encourages (via the breathing techniques) to push that energy up through the spine so that it can be distributed, filling every cell throughout the entire body. The sexual energy harnessed is not one that seeks a temporary release, but one that seeks a permanent fulfilment of something deeper that the physical body craves.

In Tantra, it is necessary to address all aspects of basic human form. Those areas are innate needs, such as food, water, movement, and sex. This does not mean that tantra (and its tantric massages) address every form. It merely means that it focuses on a form that is truly abandoned in many aspects (the sexual and spiritual form) and provides for it an outlet so that those who seek true and unadulterated health can finally find fulfilment in all of the areas.

However, you do not have to have an imbalance of any sort in order to truly enjoy a tantric massage. While it is greatly beneficial to those who suffer, it is also beneficial to those who wish to make sure that their bodies stay aligned with the universe. A tantric massage allows those who are shut off in their sexual lives to explore their sexual desires, enhance further sexual experiences, as well as become more comfortable with their sexuality in general. In the tantric belief system, the prevailing idea is that humans were created to be uninhibited beings, and that society, with its norms and its inherent guilts for things that are deemed "uncouth," have created inhibitions that we weren't naturally supposed to encounter and deal with. Tantric massages offer the option to be able to get rid of those inhibitions and flush those guilts out of our system so that we can become the being we were always meant to be.

As Tantra has evolved, it has drawn very steep correlations between those who are sick and ill and the stipulations and stressors that society constantly bombards us with. The idea is that, even though there were diseases that ran rampant for centuries before this, that studies have shown that those diseases were physically rooted in viruses and tangible reasons. They teach that many of these psychological disabilities and chronic diseases have arisen with the add-ons and pressures of a morphing society, and that this alone has created a worldwide energy imbalance when attempting to connect to the life-force of the universe.

In other words: God (or gods) have created our bodies to experience intense sexual pleasure, and it makes no sense for that to be a part of our existence that is deprived simply because a society has deemed it "inappropriate." Think about it: what if nourishing yourself with food was somehow deemed inappropriate. What if society began to teach that taking in as little food as possible would somehow make you a more acceptable person in society? There would be immense outrage as well as thousands of scientific studies pulled from the shadows as to how this trend is going to wreak havoc on the human population.

And yet, it has been done to the needed sexual aspect of being human for decades.

Utilizing a tantric massage to awaken the seven energy centres that are cantered in various positions along the spine (which have been proven to exist because of the way our major nerve centres are set up along the body's spinal cord) can lead to overall sexual health, self-awareness, treatment for many chronic aches and pains, as well as provide coping mechanisms that can serve an individual well out in society. Focusing on the purely sexual aspect of a tantric massage and deeming it inappropriate is just as close-minded as taking a look at hunting and deeming it inappropriate for everyone because you, personally, feel that hunting one's own meat is somehow inhumane.

A tantric massage has incredible benefits as well as freeing aspects that absolutely everyone can benefit from. If you can cast aside your skewed ideas of what you, personally, believe a tantric massage to be, it is possible for a client to obtain an entirely different level of existing. It can also give someone a different lens through which to view the world, as well as a way to cope with past traumas that have prevented them from having fulfilling aspects of their own individual lives. A tantric massage is a healing venture, not a sexual one. Just as society has bastardized several natural aspects of life, so it has bastardized the idea of a tantric massage.

The only true way you will ever be able to talk about it educationally is if you study up on the beliefs and then experience one.

Chapter Six:

How Do You Know it's For You?

For many people, simply deciding whether or not a tantric massage is for them is hard enough. Many people are deterred by the sexual aspect, while some people are deterred simply because they might not feel they have enough control. For eliminating these worries, research is key. Many professional and opinionated articles have been written over the years on tantric massages, and their step-by-step encounters can put the element of surprise to rest. Some people are uncomfortable with the sexual aspect of the encounter, and with that comes this proclamation: you have control over everything. From areas of the body that are touched and remain untouched all the way down to the scent of oil used to help skin glide against skin, your word is law in a tantric massage just as it is in any other massage.

Many people enjoy the fact that a tantric massage enables them to ignite passion back into their relationships. Whether it's rejuvenation in your workplace relationships because of your overall improved health and emotional state, or whether it's an improved sexual connection with your lover, the benefits far outweigh the emotional and mental insecurities that go into what someone "believes" a tantric massage to be.

Nevertheless, it doesn't stop people from worrying, and some people need bullet-pointed questions to ask themselves in order to figure out if something is right for them.

So, if you are new to the idea of a tantric massage, and you are not sure whether or not it is right for you, then here are some things you can ask yourself that will better prepare you for the decision you face:

1. Do your research. Knowing what to expect can mean the difference between an educated opinion and an opinion based on society's definitions. If you base your decisions on society's interpretation of things, it will almost always steer you wrong. Society is intentionally skewed to sell product, dictate different forms of beauty, and keep us in boxes that enable the world to run on a smoother plane. Being confident in understanding what is coming aids in the settling of the mind as well as give someone the confidence to walk in and talk informatively about their experience before it begins.

2. Once you have educated yourself on the matter, consider booking a dual massage with a friend or someone you closely trust. This can provide a delicate experience where you are delving into new territory with someone at your side, and it can help eliminate the vulnerability that might be keeping you from something like this. Enjoying something like this with someone at your side will not only create a diminished sense of vulnerability, it gives you someone to converse with after the experience, which is ideal for people who need to talk through their emotions afterward a specific experience.

3. Tantric massages are especially wonderful for aches and pains. If you are someone who suffers from daily wear and tear due to your job, or because of health issues, a tantric massage is just for you. Because of the elongated massage time and the attention to each and every

muscle, aches and pains are addressed on a muscle fibre level that traditional massages don't reach. If you have chronic headaches or migraines, the improved blood circulation because of the excessive attention given to your body means longer-lasting effects after the massage is completed. You will be able to go longer in between bouts of pain, and the massage will be able to address them on a deeper level.

4. A tantric massage is also wonderful for sexual exploration. Yes, a tantric massage has a sexual side, and there is nothing to be afraid of. For those that are wanting to explore sexually, but not sure where to start, a tantric massage is a trusting, relaxing, and controlled environment to do such exploring. It is available for both men and women, and both genders can request any gender they wish to administer the massage. You can openly control the level at which the sensuality takes place, and you can open your world to different sexual explorations while deeply thinking on other avenues you might wish to take.

5. A tantric massage is a great way to ease one's mind. Because of the sheer length of the massage and the relaxation breathing techniques and strokes involved, this kind of massage is the best at melting away stress and easing the mind from the whirlwinds of life. The safe and controlled environment helps to ease the body and mind further by providing a place that the client feels secure in during their relaxation, and this enables them to drop their guard further so they might enjoy the experience more. And, for those that have a hard time dropping their guard, a tantric massage is a great way to attempt to begin that process.

6. Another way to ease one's mind before the massage is to actively talk to the masseuse before the massage takes place. They are more than willing to answer questions, talk you through the process, ask you about any add-ons (such as hot stones or incense to aid in relaxation), and address any fears and concerns you might have. This is when you can address what you want to avoid, and you can rest assured that the professional and certified masseuse will adhere to your every word.

7. A tantric massage is for you if you simply need a way to relax. Many people view relaxation in different ways: some people enjoy a hot tub, some people enjoy a long shower, and some people enjoy intimate moments with others. You can have versions of all of these things in a tantric massage. Hot stones can be utilized to warm you from head to toe, incense and body oils can be employed to give you the feel of slickness running against your skin, and the intimate setting can provide intimacy between you and the masseuse, with yourself, or even with whomever you've decided to obtain the massage with.

Tantra is an experience born from thousands of years of religious ritual and body therapy. The bio-energy principles that it employs makes it not only a physical benefit, but a spiritual benefit as well. It's versatility to aid in emotional and mental issues makes it the ideal form of natural treatment for many different ailments, and even the healthy individual can benefit from its sheer relaxation techniques. It implores elements of a regular massage, hot stone massage, deep tissue massage, reflexology, and Indian head massages to create a whole-body experience that doesn't leave any part of the client neglected. And the best part (as well as the greatest misunderstood aspect) is that there is absolutely no sexual contact with the masseuse.

Just like any other massage, a tantric massage will involve the masseuse asking you to strip down to at least your underwear and then requiring you to cover with a sheet. Then, only the parts of the body that are being massaged will be exposed at any given time to the air of the room and the masseuse. The verbal interaction before, during, and after the massage will all remain strictly confidential, and your masseuse is nothing but a guide through the tantric ideas of relaxation, as well as its breathing techniques. They are your tour guide through this journey of relaxation, internal healing, and comfortable vulnerability, and at any point in time you can tell them when something is making you uncomfortable, and they will adjust accordingly.

Even the types of touches are under your control in a tantric massage. If something is too light, or too harsh, all you have to do is communicate that to the masseuse. But, the communication is imperative. Just as the masseuse is coaching you lightly through specific breathing techniques to enhance the experience, your communication with what you need from the masseuse will only work to deepen your overall experience, as well as your bond with the giver of the massage. A tantric massage can be a way to validate yourself as a breathing, sensual, strong being, but communication is key throughout the session.

Many people have come to believe that a tantric massage is inherently erotic because of the option to massage areas that are deemed "sexual." Massaging of the breasts, genitals, and buttocks are not unheard of in sessions like these, and many of those touches can make people uncomfortable because we have not only misconstrued the idea of sexuality, we have imprinted into our minds that touching those areas automatically constitutes sexual advances.

Think of it this way: when you are washing yourself down in a shower, is the massaging of the soap over your breasts or genitals inherently sexual? Do you find yourself scolding yourself in the shower because you touched your more sexualized areas? Of course not, that's silly. The obvious barrier is someone else doing the touching. We automatically begin to believe that someone is making sexual advances when they are touching those more intimate parts because we have been conditioned to think that way, regardless of the actual intent. It's why many women and men request the same sex doctor when they go in for their physicals. There is something inherently ingrained into us that has dictated that if someone of the opposite sex is touching our intimate areas, it is sexual and should be avoided at all costs.

This ideal not only demonizes the touching of intimate areas for purposes other than sexual, but it also demonizes sexual ideals altogether.

These two concepts work in tandem to completely ostracize an area of relaxation massage that can be more beneficial and much more stimulating (and no, not in a sexual way). Focusing merely on the "sexual" aspect and letting every other aspect fall to the wayside boils down something positive, intrinsically necessary, and incredibly bonding into something lewd, crude, and taboo. A sexual massage (which is what everyone thinks of when they hear the words "tantric" and "massage") is where receiving genital stimulation is expected to reach sexual release. A tantric massage is about losing all of those expectations so that you can inwardly reflect, become more self-aware, and enjoy the body you have been given in the moment. You can discover profound and new ways to become vulnerable, as well as centre yourself in ways you haven't ever been able to.

All you have to do is disassociate sexual aspects that you believe take place from the reality of an actual tantric massage. For men, the learn to be receivers instead of constant givers, allowing them to explore the relaxation and soothing feelings that come with being able to lean back and not have to worry about the reciprocation that is required of a male in order to not seem "cold" and "selfish." Women are sometimes people that go with the flow and hardly bring their opinions to light, and a tantric massage gives them a way to practice expressing what they want and don't want. They become more in tune with their own natural rhythms, and they slowly learn that doing things for others does not mean neglecting themselves in the process.

Therapeutic massages segments the body into good and bad zones: good zones are massaged and bad zones are strayed away from. Whole body (tantric) massages celebrate the entire body while erasing lines of shame in the process. It enables someone to become proud of their body and secure in their emotional states, and it allows them to open their world to new sensations, understandings, and connections with the world and energies around them. If you struggle with chronic pains, wish for relaxation, want to explore something new, want to become more self-aware, or want to tap into unexplored sensual desires and emotions, than a tantric massage is the right choice for you.

Chapter Seven:

Techniques and Types

There are different techniques utilized in tantric massages, no matter the type you ask for. There are some people who seek out a tantric massage as a means of sexual therapy. This type of massages aids the client in overcoming post-traumatic stress disorders that come with sexual trauma, as well as any anxieties over instilled fears of vulnerability. During this massage, there is much more communication than normal. The masseuse will be constantly reading body language as well as asking the client for feedback, and the moment the client becomes uncomfortable the massage progresses no further. However, the masseuse will not back off. They will continue on their journey unless the client specifically tells them that they are done.

Not only that, but there is heavy communication before and after the massage. The masseuse sits down with the client beforehand and discusses anything and everything that the client wishes. Then, at the end, the masseuse talks them through what happened, listens to any emotions the client is wanting to share that might have popped up in the session, and talks through the positive aspects of booking another massage. Tantric massages for sexual therapy occurs over many sessions, and is usually done with one masseuse in particular in order to aid the trust-building exercises it imposes. And, as always, these conversations are kept completely confidential.

Tantric massages can also aid men in addressing premature ejaculation. The relaxation techniques employed as well as the breathing exercises that are coached by the masseuse aid in men becoming more in sync with their bodies, enabling them to explore the aspect of better control over their pelvic regions. By tapping into their ability to receive pleasure without any regard on having to return it, it allows them the mental capacities to address the issues that are stemming the premature ejaculation.

Sexual therapy, in general, is a practice that came to fruition all the way back in the 1600s. Back then, pelvic massages were often done by physicians and midwives for many different reasons, from trying to get a woman to relax during labour all the way down to treating "female hysteria," which was a catch-all medical term for women who suffered from emotional outbursts, different sexual appetites, and anxiousness. Sexual therapy has since undergone tremendous transformations. Now, it is referred to as complement medical treatment of sexual dysfunctions when no physiological reasons exists for the issue at hand. Things addressed in this type of therapy range from premature ejaculation all the way to sexual addiction and issues with consummation.

However, within the sex therapy world, there are strict rules between exercises that can be accomplished in session between couples and what can be assigned to a single person as a requirement for treatment outside of a session. This is why tantric massages have become so popular alongside sex therapy sessions: it can address various sexual dysfunctions and mental inhibitions while staying in line with every single rule involved that regulates sex therapy on a medical level.

Many institutions, such as religious and educational ones, still find the practice of sex therapy highly controversial.

However, undergoing sexual therapy requires everything that is necessary for undergoing "regular" therapy. When someone books an appointment, the first thing that is required is a doctor recommendation that the issues being struggled with are not physiologically-based. Then, a routine evaluation is filled out, just as if an individual was seeking mental health therapy. This is to determine where the client's mindset is at, where their apprehensions lie, and what their experiences have been with the issue they are seeking help for.

In the U.S., there is an association entitled the American Association of Sex Educators, Counsellors, and Therapists (AASECT), and they are the board that oversees clinical training for people who want to be certified as sex therapists (CST). Any licensed mental health and social care worker can go through the program to become certified, and it is becoming more and more common among social workers to have this certification because of the rise in sexually traumatized children that enter their care. In these sex therapy sessions, the focus is tailored towards the symptoms being experienced rather than jumping right into the psychodynamic conflicts. This reassures the client that the professional is understanding of their issues, and the sessions then progress at the pace of the client and how they wish to divulge information. The reason for that is because any misunderstanding that the therapist might have can have dire consequences on the session, such as creating a barrier between them and the client or creating an environment of distrust.

There are many that believe the slow rise in accepting sexual therapy as a legitimate practice is what has led tantric massages to become a legitimate form of coping with sexual trauma as well as safely exploring sexual boundaries. There are thousands of positive reviews of people who have utilized tantric massages as a way to improve their sexual dysfunctions, cope with issues in their pasts, as well as enhance their overall sex life and sexual experiences.

The other form of tantric massage comes in the form of pure enjoyment. Whether it is sought professionally or experienced with another person, it is the sexual side of the experience that can come into play that rings true here. In a professional massage, there is no coping with any experiences or exploring sexual issues, there is merely relaxation, enjoyment, and the letting go of stressors and barriers as the client explores themselves inwardly while outwardly receiving a very thorough treatment. During a professional massage, breathing techniques are talked through to help enhance the experience and different massaging techniques are employed as the client asks.

The reason why many different techniques aren't employed in a tantric massage that is geared towards coping is because the focus is truly inward. Adding other components to think about reduces the amount of time the client has to reflect, cope with, and eventually attempt to overcome traumas and emotions that come with that trauma. With massages that are purely for relaxation reasons, different types of strokes and devices can be employed during the session. In these types of sessions, the masseuse is trained in various types of massages: deep tissue strokes, hot stone usage, proper essential oil treatments, as well as reflexology. Just like in the sexual trauma and dysfunction massage, communication will take place beforehand in order to establish the types of techniques the client wants to explore, and a conversation after the massage will take place to sort through emotions and provide feedback.

However, when tantric massages are employed between two individuals who are doing it to enhance their sexual realm and achieve a deeper, more sensual connection with one another, it becomes less about technique and more about safety. In professional environments, or even regulated therapeutic environments, the safety aspect is less about enforcing and more about accommodating. With personal tantric massages, safety is very much about enforcing. Communication and trust is imperative to making sure both parties stay safe, and any sort of protection that the couple feels is necessary should be employed. While tantric massages provide absolutely no focus on orgasm and sexual intimacy in the belief behind it, one also cannot ignore the road that it might prompt two people to travel down.

Make sure you understand your partner. Make sure you have free and open lines of communication. Make sure your partner understands what makes you comfortable and uncomfortable, and make sure you set out your expectations beforehand. This is not something to try with someone you have not known for very long, and the need here is to make sure that both parties understand where this is eventually heading. A tantric massage is based off of the idea of creating a deep, sensual connection with your partner while the two of you create a personal bond with the universal energies surrounding your bodies. If the goal is to orgasm, it won't be administered or experienced properly.

Communication, whether in a personal or professional setting, it key to the overall idea of safety within tantric massages. However, this does not mean that people who are bad at communicating cannot have tantric massages. Professional masseuses are professionals at reading body language, so they will be able to prompt from time to time if they watch one of their client's tense up. Experiencing a tantric massage with someone who knows you well also enables them to be able to read your body language a bit better than everyone else's, so they will be able to prompt you as well should they feel you getting uncomfortable. However, it needs to be understood that the lines of communication between masseuse and receiver need to always be open.

Many professional tantric masseuses find their clients via word of mouth. A particular professional masseuse in New York finds that her usual clients are a crowd of 9-5 workers that span some of the most stressful jobs this planet has to offer. From doctors and nurses to housewives of multiple children and teachers, she has serviced them all, and is happy to report that over 80 percent of her clientele return at least once for another massage. She says that she makes it a point to be kind, generous, and open with her clients if she expects them to be as such. She recalls one case that stood out to her very vividly. It was a woman in her 50s that began seeing her after her divorce. She proclaimed that her ex-husband had always put her down, especially when it came to their sex life. She said her insecurities spawned from the weight she had gained, and that her ex-husband used to use that against her because of his own insecurities with his impotence.

This woman ended up becoming a regular of the professional's, and has found an enhanced version of life that streams all the way into her professional work. Her co-workers have asked her time and time again why she always glows and is so happy, and the divorced-woman-in-her-50s attributes it all to her tantric masseuse and the boundaries she helped her overcome in the process.

This professional masseuse out of New York says she has been told many times that her massages were absolutely critical to the journey they were on. She admits that she hasn't had many clients that come in just for the craving of a massage. She testifies that over 90 percent of her clients come in with something they want to conquer, and that their research (as well as the raves of their friends) pushed them in this direction. After all, a tantric massage doesn't just involve a massage, it gives individuals a safe space to express their true emotions for a certain event or person without the atmosphere of being judged or "run over" with something that was more traumatizing to someone else. It gives these clients a place to safely relive, and then relieve, themselves of the pain they have been experiencing.

No matter the types of massage strokes employed, and no matter the reason why a tantric massage is being sought by the client, the same two principles apply: orgasm is never the focus, and balance between your body and the universe is essential. A tantric massage is there to enable the body to release its worries and stresses so that it can find its cosmic balance within the universe, and the consequences of that are an enhanced form of living. Where someone chooses to place that enhancement is up to them, but the important thing is that the energies flowing throughout the body are now unimpeded upon.

That is the true technique and type of tantric massage: the type that connects you with the life force of the universe.

Chapter Eight:

Keeping Tantric Massages and Sex Healthy

As we stated earlier, the key to keeping tantric massages healthy, no matter if the nature is professional or personal, is communication. The masseuse always needs to know where you stand emotionally, mentally, and physically because it helps them to gain a better understanding of what you enjoy and what relaxes you. The open lines of communication also aid to establish a connection for when the receiver becomes uncomfortable or hits an emotional barrier that they need time processing. The masseuse is not just a provider of a massage and relaxation, they are there as a professional (or personal) sounding board for emotional walls that might be hit during the course of the massage.

With a personal massage, the same rules apply. Make sure that both (or more) parties understand where it is ultimately headed. If it is just a massage, make sure all parties involved understand that. If it is going to progress beyond a massage, make sure you have proper sexual protection, such as condoms, dental dams, and spermicide, beforehand. Keeping yourself physically safe when utilizing something as freeing as a tantric massage is an absolute must.

During a professional tantric massage, a shower is usually taken by the client. This is an extra step of protection for both parties, ensuring that nothing can be exchanged between the two parties. A safe and relaxed environment is provided, and any add-ons that the client might want is talked about beforehand so that the receiver of the massage can think less on what is coming and more on the relaxation that is to be had. The breathing techniques that the masseuse will coach the client through is to help when anxiousness arises, not just to help relax the client. When anxiousness happens, knee-jerk reactions can occur, and the breathing techniques help to build a wall between the two reactions and prompt healthy and proper discussion of what is going on.

Another way that a professional keeps themselves safe during tantric massages is the use of rubber gloves when massaging areas of the body that are considered more sensitive. This enables them to lower their risk of being exposed to sexually transmitted issues, as well as protects the client from being exposed to any residual oils and bacteria's that might be on the hands of the masseuse after the bulk of the massage has been completed. Another safety point is that, at any point in time, you can stop the massage or tell the masseuse to skip a part of your body that you might not feel comfortable massaging.

Staying safe and healthy while utilizing a tantric massage for your own benefits stems from keeping a few common sense rules in the forefront of your mind: use protection if you believe the massage might gravitate towards a sexual encounter, never engage or perform a tantric massage on someone you do not know well, and always keep the lines of communication open (both positive and negative) between all parties involved. If necessary, read and research on how to interpret body language. The truth of the matter is that some people are not very good at communication, and their bodies will tell you more than their mouths will. To bridge that gap, it is the responsibility of the masseuse to keep a strong eye out for any inclinations (such as tensing muscles and unnecessary moving) that point towards the receiver of the massage becoming uncomfortable.

A tantric massage is a wonderful way to stay healthy. It promotes inward assessment, emotional settlement, mental acuity, and physical relaxation. In a world that constantly tries to time-manage in order to squeeze the last bit of productivity we can from every single minute, it becomes harder and harder as a society to put an emphasis on relaxation and self-care. A tantric massage lumps many different forms of self-care into one three-hour massage. In a way, it tailors itself to society by harnessing and addressing multiple issues at once, and in another way it bucks against society by forcing you to slow down for such a long period of time in order to focus on yourself and what you need.

Within the beliefs that prompt the religious idea and ritual of tantric massages, it recognizes that ordinary sex prompts the body to tense. As orgasm approaches, the muscles contract, actively attempting to force the orgasm to light. This promotes aches, pains, cramps, and can even contribute to pulled muscles. Now, while this idea of sex might be very appealing to some, for many it is just a means to an end. The beliefs behind a tantric massage promote relaxation and allowing emotional and physical sensations to slowly wash over your body. The massage promotes relaxation, the breathing techniques promote emotional enjoyment, and the connection you harness between yourself and the universe around you aid in the ability to allow your body to fully experience things without your psychological parameters and blockades interfering.

Utilizing a tantric massage as a wellness check-up is something that many returning customers do. The average returning customer indulges in a tantric massage twice a month in order to make sure their physical, emotional, and mental energies are all aligned. It is not just used as a time to relax, but a time to inwardly reflect. Some people use it as a safe and secure environment to let their minds wander about work and the career trajectory they are on, and some people use the healthy environment as a way to reflect on their families. Some people utilize it as their "me time," enabling them to focus inwardly on unresolved emotions or situations that they feel need to be case aside, and some people even encourage their friends to come have a joint tantric massage with them because they derive relaxation and happiness from showcasing their secrets to others.

However any one person focuses themselves for a tantric massage is solely up to the individual. No two tantric massages are alike, and many people end up requesting the same person over and over because of a trust that builds over time. A professional tantric masseuse doesn't just become someone who provides a well-rounded massage, they become an unbiased sounding board for those intimate thoughts that someone is scared they might be judged for. It isn't just the massage that is the benefit, it is also the conversations before and after that people crave. There are many people that admit to having a tantric massage solely for the conversations that take place, because in a world where judgement is constantly around every corner, being able to find a place to sound off without being criticized is rare... And it is something that many people find they crave without ever realizing it.

While a tantric massage is not for everyone, it is something that should be experienced at least once by every single person on this planet. The energies that it can centre and the self-awareness that it can promote is something that many people need in this purely physical society that is being bred. Those that believe a tantric massage is just a legal form of a "happy ending" massage have already succumbed to the mere physicality that the massage promotes. Comparing a tantric massage to a "happy ending" massage is like comparing a girl who has a school crush on a professor to a student who is actually having sex with a professor. That professor is there to teach, guide, and settle the mind of the student while expanding their knowledge and broadening their options for their lives. A student having sex with a professor is just that: engaging in something sexual while doing something illegal... Just like a "happy ending" massage.

A tantric massage is something that is utilized to broaden the perspective of one's mind, expand the knowledge of the universe as any one individual sees it, and guide the client (or partner) through relaxation-engaging breathing techniques that aid in the overall experience of becoming inwardly synced with one's body and emotions instead of consistently neglecting them. If a sexual pleasure comes because of the massage strokes, that is purely coincidental, just like the girl with the school crush. Obviously, if the tantric massage is being experienced between two lovers, these boundaries don't always occur. But, in a professional setting, that is the difference... And it is a *massive* one that needs to be understood in a society that has skewed and boiled it down to one specific purpose: sex.

Tantric massages are healthy, relaxing, and promote the cantering of one's energies and soul among the universe. They come with many of the proven health benefits that come with regular massages, as well as some health benefits that aren't always achieved in regular massages. The beliefs within Tantra are physically manifested within tantric massages, and the principles that Tantra teaches are physically manifested within the after-effects of a properly administered one.

Release your preconceptions, embrace the realities, and look within yourself to find what you truly need. And, if you need help doing that? Then, a tantric massage is just what you are looking for.

www.ingramcontent.com/pod-product-compliance
Lightning Source LLC
Chambersburg PA
CBHW071251280526
45788CB00004B/1670